I0410471

Pei

Thermal Zone System

By

Fath Saelock

1663 LIBERTY DRIVE, SUITE 200
BLOOMINGTON, INDIANA 47403
(800) 839-8640
WWW.AUTHORHOUSE.COM

First published by AuthorHouse 10/09/04

ISBN: 1-4208-0148-1 (sc)

Printed in the United States of America
Bloomington, Indiana

This book is printed on acid-free paper.

Dear Readers,

This is a letter of apology. Prior to writing this book, I have distributed some business cards proclaiming myself as a doctor. Even thought in my opinion I deserve to be called a doctor, I have no right to called myself one. I haven't gone through the proper schooling to earn my degree. Although there is no school that teaches such a revolutionary health system, it is not an excuse for what I have done. I apologize if I have misled and/or offended anyone for my past action. I will leave it up to the readers to decide whether or not I am worthy to be a Doctor of Chinese Healing.

Sincerely,
Fath Saelock

Acknowledgement

I am dedicating this book to my late father, Fong Saelock. Thanks to him I received this ancient Chinese healing secret. I don't know how he learned about it but I'm sure he wants me to share it with the world. It is not easy to convince the world about the ultimate cure, the body itself.

I would also like to thank a colleague of mine, John Reaves, he believed, stood by me, and supported my dream. I would also like to thank Priscilla Franco for editing this book and Kent Huang for the design work. It has really meant a lot to me. In addition, I would like to thank my family and best friends for understanding and lending their moral support instead of criticism. I could not have written this book without their support. I have tried to have someone else write this book, but I came to realize that nobody understands the system better than I do. In the past, I always relied on others to fulfill my dream, but everyone has their own dream, ambition, and agenda. I understand now that if I really want this book to be written, I must write it myself. Even now I can not believe that I am an author.

Table of Contents

Philosophy

The body is the **one and only true cure to all illnesses** caused either by nature and/or by us. No doctors or physicians to date have healed or cured any symptomatic, causative, and/or chronic illnesses. The best that can be done is to create the best condition whereby the body can heal itself without hindrance. Every treatment is either aiding or hindering the body's healing ability. Illnesses (symptomatic) that occur overnight can be cured by the body overnight and illnesses (chronic) that are caused by years of abuse and/or neglect to the body require years to reverse (cure). Diseases can only exist in a weak body with poor immunity; they can not exist in a strong and healthy body. Like the saying goes, "the best defense is a strong offense." You must keep the body strong so it can attack first rather than waiting to be attacked and then defend itself. We are living in a cesspool of germs and viruses which can change and mutate. Without the body's immune system to fight sickness and disease mankind wouldn't able to survive long. We must fight fire with fire. *The body's healing ability can be imitated but never duplicated.* This is not my system or anyone else's system but it is the body's system. **The body will heal itself**

or you won't get well. This is the Pei Thermo-Zone System slogan. The Pei Thermal Zone System is a very unique system that does not require anyone's opinion to validate it nor does it predicated on one's belief.

About the body

We tend to forget that we are warm blooded human beings and that cold in any form is the body's worse enemy. The human body is complete and is designed to function as a unit. Each body part or organ has its own function and purpose in life. Each body part and organ work together and rely on each other to keep the body in top condition. Loss of any body part or organ makes the body incomplete and will result in health problems in the future.

The human body is not like Frankenstein's body with interchangeable body parts or organs. Whatever we are born with that is all we have. Replacement body parts and organs can never perform and function as well as the original. The compatibility is the major problem facing people who have transplants. Those born with abnormalities do not choose this but may require assistance. However, the majority of us have no excuse to abuse and neglect the body intentionally and then complain.

There are several organs and body parts that directly affect the blood which are the key elements that make this system work. The key elements are blood, the naval, digestive track, small intestine, lungs, and the hand. Not to say the rest of the body is unimportant, but only a few organs and body parts directly affect the blood.

The first and most important organ is the blood. I remember something that John has taught me. He said **life itself is in the blood**. It is blood that connects and gives life to the rest of the body. Like a computer (body), there are many components (organs and body parts) but without electricity (blood) to power the computer, it (body) is as good as dead. The second body part we need to acknowledge is the naval. There is a saying, "the eyes are the windows to the soul." Since that's the case **the naval is the doorway to life.** Inside our mother's womb we are connected to life support through the naval. The naval also act as the thermostat that regulates the body's temperature. So protecting the naval from the cold is a very important task because the blood's number one enemy is the cold. The third is the digestive track which processes the foods and water and turns it into energy and body heat. It is the digestive process that gives the blood all the nutrients it needs. The fourth organ is the small intestine where all the waste is stored and waits for disposal. Sooner or later, like the saying goes, "what goes in must come out." If foods are left in the body too long, it becomes toxic (waste) and poisons the blood. The fifth organ we need to point out is the lung. The blood needs oxygen to survive and only the lung can provide it. That is why the lungs are so important. The last body part we must acknowledge is the hand. It is the hand that protects the naval from exposure to cold and heat. Without the hand there will be no technique which the Pei System is based upon. **Notice how everything revolves around the blood**.

Scenario 1:

You got a nasty cut preparing dinner. You stop the bleeding but you lose a lot of blood in just minutes. You start to get lightheaded and feel a little dizzy. You stop whatever you were doing and just lay down so the body can recover the blood you just lost. The rest of the family is about to be home and you don't have the energy to continue cooking dinner because you too are hungry. You went to the fridge and ate the leftovers without heating it up. As you were eating, you could feel energy coming back to you. The body has the sufficient nourishment it needs to produce energy for you to finish cooking dinner in the nick of time.

Scenario 2:

You just had an operation to remove one of your kidneys. The doctor says you can survive with just one kidney. A couple years later, the other kidney is about to give out because of the level of abuse inflicted on the kidneys remains the same. There is only one kidney handling twice the work of filtering toxins. Yes you can survive with just one kidney but your quality of life will always be less than before. You change your lifestyle and take better care of yourself and hope for a donor. The wait for a donor is very long and the thought of you missing a kidney makes you feel incomplete, like there is a void inside of you. You make sure you don't abuse your body anymore because the next time it might not be only your kidney that is failing you.

Scenario 3:

You got injured while playing a routine football game with friends. You took a strong pain killer to numb the pain so you can continue playing. It seems that finishing the game is more important than your own health. You cannot go to sleep the whole night because of the pain. You were in so much pain that you can't even get up out of bed. You could continue masking the pain by taking more painkillers or just rest more so the body has time to heal itself. You called in sick at work and rested for the day without taking drugs. The pain lessened enough for you return to work the very next day.

Introduction

The Pei Thermal-Zone System is a revolutionary ancient Chinese healing secret. This system is unique because for the first time ever the body's true healing potential is finally unleashed and realized. *The system maximizes the body's healing ability; if there is a cure, the body will reveal it.* I have witnessed many people from all walks of life and cultures use the technique without really knowing what they are doing and the healing properties associated with the technique. We are so close to the answer yet so far away. The cure is literally under our nose, no wonder we missed it. This system is the exception to the rule," if it sounds too good to be true, therefore it is not true." It is because of the simplicity of the system that boggles the human mind. This book will open up your mind and help you think in a whole new light. A common sense approach combined with logical science will astound you. You will be amazed at the simplicity of the system.

Ambient temperature

Ambient temperatures are atmospheric and environmental temperatures that affect the body. In other words, it is Mother Nature's temperature which we have no control over. We must take precautions and protect ourselves from the ever changing weather. We cannot control the weather but we can change the ambient temperature to a certain point. We tend to always find ways of changing the ambient temperature around our body instead of changing the body's internal temperature.

Scenario 4:

You are out camping with a couple friends. It is a chilly night and you need to start a fire to cook dinner. You sit close to the flame because the heat from the fire warms you up. After the meal, you and your friends sit around the camp fire for story telling and add more wood to the fire when it dies down. It is time to hit the sack and you decided to sleep near the fire in a sleeping bag rather than leave the warm camp fire to sleep in a cold tent. The camp fire warms up the ambient heat so you don't feel the chill throughout the night.

Scenario 5:

You are home and it is cold but you don't want to run up the electricity bill by turning on the heater to warm the entire house. You start up the fire place and burn a couple pieces of logs in the living room. It is getting late and you decided to call it a night. You head up to your bedroom to find it is freezing so you turn on the portable electric heater and the room slowly warms up. You woke up feeling stuffy because there is no air circulation in your room. You got up and cracked open the window just a little for fresh air. You got back to bed and woke up in the morning to find the room is chilly rather than warm. Because you were under heavy blankets, the cold doesn't bother you until you get up from under the covers.

Scenario 6:

You are invited to a big party and there will be a lot of people. It is a cold night and you wore a thick jacket. When you got to the party you felt hot. You asked the hosts if they turned on the heater and their reply was no. You look around and see a lot of dancing and sweating going on. Then you figure it out, it is all those bodies giving out heat in a house with few openings for ventilation. You step outside to get fresh air and you take off your jacket before you head back into the party. The ambient temperatures are extremely cold outside while it is extremely hot indoors.

Chap 1: Temperature Chaos

In order to maintain body heat, you must first understand what causes it and how to control it. Ambient temperature is everywhere and different from place to place. The body adjusts its internal temperature to accommodate the ambient temperature the naval is reading. When the naval senses a sudden change of ambient temperature from extreme heat to extreme cold and vice versa, the body will raise or lower its temperature to reach its equilibrium (optimal body heat). The body becomes confused and starts rising and lowering its temperature creating a fluctuation of body temperature. This state of instability of the body's temperature is referred to as Temperature Chaos.

The body's natural state is balancing its internal temperature by controlling temperature chaos. The body know how to self regulate its own temperature so it will never over or under heat itself. We are taught that 98.6° f is the body's normal temperature which means based on the Pei System it is the body's equilibrium temperature. I can't say that this is true because the body fluctuates all the time and to pinpoint an exact temperature in my opinion is wrong. Nobody can really pinpoint the equilibrium temperature except the body itself. The equilibrium range is very narrow and very hard to hit the mark. You can be at the equilibrium range but that is simply a rough estimate not the exact equilibrium. The body radiates heat nonstop 24 hours a day, 7 days a week and how we retain and maintain the body's heat will determine ones' health and well being. Maintaining the body's temperature at its equilibrium range helps the body's ambient temperature transition itself from hot to cold and vice versa. Just like your eyes need transition from light to dark and vice versa, the body needs to transition itself to prevent any temperature shock. If the body's temperature is slightly above or under the equilibrium range the body is considered to be affected by temperature chaos. When does the body reach equilibrium? Nobody really knows for sure except the body itself.

Temperature chaos is an equal opportunist predator that preys on every human being. We never gave it (fluctuation of body heat) a name in the past so we do not know how to prevent it until now. Every illness is directly or indirectly related with the fact that the body cannot maintain equilibrium. Temperature chaos affects the blood by either heating it up or cooling it down which is bad for the body. You will be shocked to know that the body is constantly under attack by ambient temperature causing the body to be in a state of temperature chaos. Our lack of awareness about temperature chaos is what jeopardizes our own health.

I can still remember when I was attending school; my dad would always warn me to beware of a chilly but sunny day. I didn't understand what he was trying to tell me. Like a kid it enters one ear and exits another. I didn't see any significance in the technique so I didn't value it. Now that I think about it, I came to understand what he meant. In my mind I don't need to wear a jacket because it is sunny outside therefore it must be warm. As soon as I got outside, I started shaking and feeling a chill. As I was walking to school, I could feel a little warmth from the sunlight but when I walked into the shade I could feel a chill again. It is the constant switching of (warm to cold and vice versa) ambient temperature that caused me to get the sniffles the next day. These kinds of days are dangerous because it gives us a false sense of warmth so we are always ill-prepared for the cold that awaits us outside. Now I observe others making the same mistake as I did as a kid; accepting the cold and just dealing with it and hoping that the sunlight will eventually give off enough heat so you won't feel the cold anymore.

Scenario 7:

It is sunny day but when you step outside without a jacket or sweater, you feel a sudden chill throughout your body even though you are in the sunlight. You got into your car which happens to be parked in the shade. The chill intensifies for a couple of minutes until you warm up the engine and turn on the heater. When you get out of your car into the sunlight again, you feel colder then warmer. Your reasoning is that you should feel warm outside because of the sunshine, but what you don't realize is that the sunlight take awhile to warm up the ambient temperature around the naval. Next time you know better to not under estimate the weather.

Scenario 8:

It is winter time and it is extremely cold outside. You have the heat on high in your home and your body is warm.

Your friend calls and you decide to go out to dinner together. You slip on a heavy jacket and step outside. A sudden chill rushes under your jacket and cools the ambient temperature around your naval. You stand in the cold long enough and notice that the chill slowly disappears. Your body becomes more adapted to the cold and then you enter the restaurant and it is very warm. You take off your jacket because you feel hot. The sudden switch from extreme warm air to extreme cold air then back to extreme warm air shocks your body causing you to catch a cold the next day.

Scenario 9:

You are in a warm bed with a heavy blanket. Suddenly you wake up and need to use the restroom, but the room is freezing. You decided to get up anyhow because you have to go. The moment you got up from under the covers, your body's heat dissipated in a flash. The chill caused you to shake and gave you goose bumps. After you use the restroom, you get back under your blanket which is still warm. You shiver for a couple of minutes and then the chill disappears. You can't go back to sleep because your stomach is growling. You know you must get up again into the cold kitchen to eat something. During the entire time you are eating, you are shaking and thinking about being in bed under your warm blankets.

Chap. 2: RS Technique (waking hour)

This technique has been in existence for thousands of years. Many people have used this very technique for health reasons. They have used it without fully understanding how and why it worked. They use it for brief moment to feel better and stop either because they tend to forget about it or it never dawns on them that such a simple technique can do so much. I have shared this technique with many people and when I ask them if they have tried it, their response was either I forgot or it doesn't work for me. It is funny how even though the technique works, if they cannot figure out how and why it works, it doesn't work in their mind. There are some who benefit from the technique but never share it with anyone else because they don't know how to explain it to the person, or the reason to use it. I write this book as a way to explain the reason why one should use this technique.

This is the very technique my dad taught me as a kid and now I am going to share it with you. This technique is called Reaves & Sealock Technique (RS Technique) and it is very simple but effective. What you do is take the palm of your hand and place it over the naval. I recommend you do skin to skin contact, meaning your hand under your clothing. That is all there to the technique. You can use your feet and it will also work, but it is much easier and convenient to use your palm. Since the hands (extremity) are connected by blood vessels (heat), by placing your palm over the naval (thermostat), you are doing two things. The hand acts as an insulator, by insulating the naval to read ambient temperature and at the same time send the reading of the hand's temperature to the naval. The naval can then request the permission from the heart to create more than enough blood, so the excess can be sent to the extremities (hands, feet, & head). Eventually the whole body will warm up and correct any problem the body is experiencing. By shielding the naval from ambient temperature, you are preventing temperature chaos from affecting the body's internal heat source. That is why the hand is so important to this system.

Have you ever seen someone cross their arm when they feel cold? Every one does it including me when I was younger. Believe it or not, it is a universal habit. It is a natural response of the body to cross its arm when the naval senses cold. What the body really is trying to do is have the arm cover the naval and protect it from the cold. Because the arm crossed is not low enough to cover the naval, the technique is used in its place. The hand is the only extremity that can reach the naval.

The RS Technique is not only useful to help the body warm up and stay warm. It is also used to help keep the body cool during the summer. The technique helps the body by achieving and maintaining equilibrium. If the body's temperature is below equilibrium then sensitivity to heat increases; as the body temperature reaches equilibrium the sensitivity to heat decreases. For example, you took a very hot shower and the surface of your skin is hot and as long as you stay in the bathroom you don't feel the intense heat created by the steam. As soon as you step out of the bathroom, you feel cold because the surface of your skin is hot so when it comes in contact with cooler air your sensitivity to cold increases. Then when someone else with cooler (normal) skin surface walks into the bathroom still steamy, he complains it is hot. The closer your skin temperature is to the ambient heat the less heat you will feel and the less the body needs to sweat to compensate. If the body heat level passes above equilibrium then the body will cool itself down just a little by sweating.

You might ask yourself if this technique is so important to maintaining good health, why since the dawn of humanity have no doctors, physicians, or scientists come up with this technique. The reason why nobody comes up with the technique as a healing tool is because humans are always advancing in thinking. You can't find the answer if you only think inside the box. We take what exists and improve on it. The search for a cure becomes more complicated as we try to "out discover" other discoveries. The more complicated the mind gets the further we are from the answer. Like the saying goes, "the shortest distant from point A to point B is a straight line." Don't forget, "the more plumbing you add the more chance of a clog." These two sayings simply tell us that the answer is simple but we complicate everything. We take credit for discoveries which ultimately end up relying and depending on the body's healing ability. You will never find the answer if you don't give credit where credits is due. John Reaves once told of a verse in the Bible, "God takes the simple things in the world to confound the wise." I truly believe this saying because it really lends itself to this system. The simplicity of this system has all the wise and smart people overlooking it.

For most of my adult life, I have been occasionally using the technique when I remembered (which was hardly). I got mixed results since I did not use it consistently. For the last 10 years, I have been testing the technique on myself every chance I got to see if there is a limit to the body's healing ability. I literally became my own guinea pig to understand and discover the body's healing secret. I find that there is no limit to the body's healing potential provided that the body is complete, in one piece and not being abused or neglected. I shared the technique with others and they all received the same benefits. I feel better now than when I was 20 years old. In a way, I am in control of my own health.

Scenario 10:

You are planning to go out into the cold. Before you head outside you test your stomach's temperature, it is cool to the touch. You put on a sweater and a jacket to be on the safe side. You take half hour to use the RS technique to warm up your internal temperature. As you sit watching television, you can feel the heat starting to radiate in your stomach and throughout your body. When you step outside, you didn't feel a chill at all except a stinging sensation on you hands and face. The cold can penetrate the jacket and even the sweater, but the cold has a hard time penetrating the barriers of body heat (last line of defense). You remain nice and warm while your friend is shivering.

Scenario 11:

You are working in an office and it is cold because of all the computers. You run around a lot so you feel warm enough not to wear a jacket, but you have one on anyhow. You feel a little hot and instead of taking your jacket off, you take a 15 minute break to use the RS Technique to warm up your insides. After the break, the hot feeling disappears and you just feel comfortable. The barrier of body heat is retained by your jacket and that's what kept you warm not hot for the rest of the day. You feel comfortable while the rest of your co-workers are either feeling cold or hot.

Scenario 12:

It is summer and it is very hot. You don't have an option of turning on the air conditioner. You only can take a shower to stay cool. Instead of taking a cold shower like everyone else, you take a hot shower. You apply the RS technique before you get out of the shower, you can feel a cool sensation as the fan cools down your hot body. An hour later, your whole body is cool to the touch except the area around the naval which stays warm because of the technique. You continue using the technique with the fan turned on low to circulate the ambient heat from the body, while everyone complains about being hot except you.

Chap. 3: Pillow Technique (rest hour)

This is the Pillow Technique which started it all. This technique is similar to the RS Technique except it is use during sleeping hours. It is the most important technique of the two because your hands are free from doing anything. This technique helps to warm up your entire body, put you into deep sleep within an hour instead of a couple of hours. It also helps you to improve digestion for maximum energy in the morning.

You place the palm of your hand over the naval like the RS Technique. Then you put a pillow over the hand that's covering the naval and cover your entire body including the pillow with an adequate blanket. This technique is most useful during winter time when it is very cold at night. For those who toss and turn too much and the pillow never stays still, simply wear a sweater or light jacket and then use the technique while under an adequate blanket. The sweater or jacket acts as a pillow to retain the body heat except the sweater or jacket will not move. The purpose is to elevate the body's temperature with the technique so the torso or stomach (core) temperature can reach equilibrium and then maintain that temperature with a pillow, sweater, or jacket for as long as possible.

In the summer time, just use the technique and a pillow and cover the stomach with a blanket so that the pillow will not move around. You want to retain maximum heat surrounding the naval area and allow the rest of the body to be exposed so it can vent off any excess heat. Turn a fan on low to gradually circulate the ambient heat given off by the body. You will feel cooler as the fan moves the heat surrounding the body and replaces it with cool night air. If you happen to wake up in the middle of the night, check your stomach's temperature and you will realize that it is cool to the touch. The ambient heat created by the body has evaporated and has been replaced by the ambient cool or cold air of the room. Re-apply the pillow technique and you will fall back to sleep right away. This technique is very important and essential to maintaining good health. The body can not relax if it is constantly cold. You need heat if you want the body to relax especially the muscles. It may be confusing since it is already a hot day and we are warming up the body with the technique. However, the answer is simple. If the temperature of your skin is higher than the ambient room temperature due to the pillow technique, then the room's air feels cooler to you. If the body reaches equilibrium and the ambient room temperature is even higher, then the body will vent more heat through the extremities, but the stomach should still maintain equilibrium at all times. If your skin temperature is lower than the ambient room temperature due to sweating, then you will sense more heat. Without the pillow technique everyone would still curl up into the fetal position when the body senses cold.

Remember that the body goes into the fetal position to protect the stomach or torso from loosing heat. The body uses the thighs and chest to create an enclosure to retain the body's heat, so it can still be able to recover from the cold. It is a natural response of the body to go into the fetal position when cold affects the core temperature through the naval. When someone goes into the fetal position, is a good indication that temperature chaos has affected the body's core temperature. By applying the pillow technique, you help the body raise its temperature and prevent the naval from sensing any cold air. The body will not curl up if the body achieves equilibrium and you help maintain it throughout the night.

In the case of hypothermia, the body draws blood from the extremities (hands, feet, and head) to sustain the stomach's heat level because the stomach or torso has the most concentration of blood (heat). If the heat level in the stomach or torso is diminished then life (blood) itself ceases to survive. As the extremities develop frostbite or gangrene, the body parts need to be amputated or else the dead flesh will spread into the rest of the body parts.

I was like everyone who did not know what I had until I was ready. I can still remember it like yesterday, I would always kick off the blanket in the summer and my dad would put the cover back on. After a while of no success in keeping me covered, my dad made a deal with me. He told me that I did not have to cover up completely, if I agreed to put my hand over my naval and only cover the stomach with a blanket. I agreed and quickly fell asleep. Of course I did not know how important the technique was until I shared it with John. Now I understand the importance of the technique and value it greatly. This is the technique which the Pei system is all based upon.

Scenario 13:

You were asleep and woke up in the fetal position. You got up and put on another blanket and got back under the covers. You can still feel the chill and your feet are freezing. After a while you feel stuffy and hot because the blankets are too heavy and the heat is trapped with nowhere to vent the excess body heat. Luckily you knew of the technique and removed one of the blankets to prevent the body from suffocating. You applied the pillow technique and within an hour your entire body warmed up including your feet. Your entire body becomes relaxed and you can hardly stay awake even though you try. You fell asleep and woke up feeling refreshed the next morning.

Scenario 14:

You can't go to sleep because it is too hot. You are sweating too much and the fan seems to be blowing hot air instead of cool air. Your place doesn't have an air conditioner installed so you apply the pillow technique but this time you didn't use any blankets just a pillow. You can feel your stomach warming up and the fan seems to be changing from blowing hot air to blowing cool air. The cooling wind of the fan kept you at a comfortable state and you quickly fell asleep. You slept through the night without waking up and woke up refreshed in the morning.

Scenario 15:

It is very cold outside but you have the heater on high and the entire apartment is warm. You went to bed only using a thin blanket because the room is warm. You open the window a little for some fresh air because it feels stuffy. You wake up in the middle of the night and your entire body is cold to the touch. The room is so cold because the cold air is trapped in your room and never reaches the thermostat to trigger it to turn on the heat. You have the option of shutting the window completely and opening the bedroom door to the living room where the thermostat is located, or add another blanket to keep the body warm. You decided not to just add a blanket but use the pillow technique as well, and you quickly fall back to sleep.

Chap 4: Heat retainer

The body is constantly producing body heat to help the blood circulate properly. Whether the body is resting or doing something, it needs food, water, and oxygen to convert into energy and heat. The rate of body heat lost is determined by how well we help the body retain the heat it creates. It is a very simple task of keeping the body warm and yet we fail miserably. During sleep, we retain the body's heat with blankets and during waking hours we help the body retain heat by wearing more clothing.

Blankets

Every one uses blankets when they go to sleep. The blankets don't produce heat, the body does. The blanket is simply an insulator for the body. The blanket retains the body heat and releases it slowly so the body stays warm and vents off any excess body heat. What about electric heating blankets you may ask? Everyone goes to sleep cold without knowing it. The level of warmth of the body will determine whether or not you get a good night's rest. Since the body is still cold after using a blanket, many use electric heating blankets thinking that the heat created by the blanket will warm the body up. It is a bad idea because the body can't regulate the heat level generated by the blanket. This means that the electric blanket can raise the body's temperature past the equilibrium range and cause a fever or lower your temperature so you'll catch a cold. Either way the body is affected by temperature chaos. Besides it is easier to warm up from the inside out using the pillow technique then forcing the heat from the outside in. Prolong use of electric blankets can cause serious health risks.

The body needs to convert a lot of foods to generate heat. Don't believe the advice you get from doctors saying it is bad to eat something before bedtime. In the past, before the pillow technique, I understood why doctors gave such advice. The body is cold throughout the night so the foods you just ate before bedtime won't process properly, and it gets stuck in the body causing problems. This is the reason why doctors recommend that you eat early and wait a couple of hours for the body to digest some of the food before you sleep. Even though you felt hungry, you are not allowed to eat because of the fear of getting fat and health issues the doctor instills in you. You deprive the body of the nutrients it needs by ignoring the body's cry for sustenance. Take the camel for example. Camels have two humps for carrying water for a particular reason. They need lots of water because they journey long distances through the desert with only the water they can carry in their two humps. Who is to say that eating late at night is bad for you? Based on the Pei System, it is better to eat anything one hour before bed time than nothing at all. Include some meat in the diet because it gives the body long lasting energy that carries you through the long night. Let's say you finish eating no later than 8 p.m. and you do some house chores for two hours such as washing dishes and laundry which practically burns up half of the food you just ate. By the time you go to bed around 10 p.m., you are running on half empty. From 8 p.m. of the previous night to the next morning at 7 a.m., it is approximately 11 hours between refueling. Can you imagine how the body feels 11 hours later since its last meal? No wonder the body is burnt out and needs artificial stimulants in the morning such as coffee to function. You might argue that the body does not need to burn a lot of foods since it is resting. However, that is not true because the colder the days are the more the body need to burn foods for heat. Just because the body does not have activities to warrant energy, this does not mean it will not need heat. It takes a lot of foods to generate body heat. What if you eat around 10 p.m. and go to sleep at 11 p.m., you have excess food for the night. As long as you use the pillow technique when going to bed, the body will burn what it needs and carry the rest of your energy into the morning so you still feel energized before eating breakfast. Do not wait until the body is completely empty before you eat because you will feel tired and sleepy. The body needs energy to produce energy so it is wise to overlap the food. That means when you feel hungry you should eat so the body has energy left over from the previous meal to convert the current meal into more energy.

Clothing

Clothing is one of the several necessities in life. Clothing serves two purposes. It is used to cover up the flesh as well as keep the body warm. Fashion industries have changed the purpose of wearing clothing. Now clothing is worn merely for fashion statements rather than for functionality.

Everywhere you look, people are inadequately dressed for the weather. Especially woman's clothing because most of their apparel are designed with little fabric which offer little or no protection against the cold. Their motto is the more flesh showing the merrier. Clothing that exposes the naval to the harsh ambient temperatures are the rage these days. Nowadays, it is not enough to just wear a jacket or sweater because indoor and outdoor temperatures are too extreme. In the winter time it is usually too cold outside and too hot inside and vice versa in the summer. This kind of inconsistent temperature shock has many not wearing adequate clothing because it is simply too much a hassle of putting on when outdoors and taking off when indoors.

The solution is to use the RS technique and wear layered clothing. What this does is help the body raise its temperature to reach equilibrium and create layers of body heat. In order for the cold air to affect the naval, it must first penetrate the layered clothing as well as the layered body heat. Remember there is a layer of body heat between every layer of clothing you wear. The combination of the technique and the layered clothing will keep the body warm and not experience any temperature shock so you will feel comfortable no matter what kind of ambient temperature environment you are in.

Chap 5: Body Fat

Body fat is a natural insulator for the body. The body will determine how much body fat it needs. ***If you don't put on a jacket, the body will do it for you.*** The body fat serves another purpose besides insulating. It also acts as a cushion for the body because if you bumped into something, how much direct impact to the bones and vital organs is determined by how much fat you have. Too much fat is not good and neither is too little fat.

You want to know why some people have high a metabolism while others do not. The answer lies with the way the umbilical cord is cut and whether your naval intrudes in, how deep or flat it is, or if you naval extrudes out. The fat builds up everywhere on the body, primarily on the stomach, but it never builds up on the naval. Your naval stay the same no matter how much fat you accumulate. The deeper your naval intrude, the lower your metabolism is and the more important it is to use the technique to compensate. The more your naval extrudes, the higher your metabolism is and you need to use the technique as well as more clothing because you lack a natural insulator. The body fat insulates body heat but if the internal temperature is cold then it is insulating cold not heat. Think of fat like a thermos, it will insulate heat if you pour hot water in, but if you pour cold water in, it will keep the water cool. Overweight people have a lot of insulation so they seldom wear a jacket or sweater or else they feel hot. Thin people are very sensitive to cold because their skins are their only natural insulator which is not much protection, if any. That is why thin people always have to wear extra clothing everywhere they go.

Have you ever wondered why babies don't stop crying even though you fed and diapered them? When you propped baby on your shoulder, the baby calmed down and fell asleep. The reason is because your shoulder acts like a hand to insulate the baby's naval from ambient temperatures. A baby's body temperature should always be hot to the touch because they don't have a lot of body fat to insulate their tiny little bodies from the cold. A baby's entire body heat needs to be retained by wearing more clothing or adding a blanket. A baby is extremely sensitive to ambient cool or cold air so always protect the entire body not only the naval. Feel the baby's hand, if it is cool, then it safe to say the baby's stomach is also cool. By placing your hand under the covers, you warm the baby's naval until the baby's hand and feet are warm. Once the baby's body temperature reaches equilibrium range, the baby will naturally fall asleep. The same applies to the elderly. Their bodies need assistance to warm up. Although the elderly are constantly cold and wearing heavy clothing, this still does not help much. By having the elderly use the RS Technique during the day and the Pillow Technique during rest, this will help them warm up and stay warm. For ages this has remained a fact but no one really understood why until now.

Talking about RS Technique reminds me of the original Star Wars when Luke Skywalker destroyed the Death Star with one missile. I think of the torso or stomach as Death Star, the naval as the ventilation shaft leading to the core, cold air as the missile, and wind as the propulsion of the missile. The torso or stomach is heavily insulated with fat and clothing like the Death Star. The only way cold air can penetrate and affect the core temperature is through the naval, just like a missile enters the ventilation shaft to destroy Death Star from the inside out.

Scenario 16:

It is summer time and there is no air conditioning. You can't go to sleep even though the fan is blowing full blast. Your parents cover you up because they know that in the middle of the night, it is very cold. They are afraid you might catch a cold. You kick off the blanket like any kid would do. You finally fall asleep for a couple hours and are awakened by the cold. Your entire body is cold to the touch. You cover yourself but it was too late because when you woke up the next morning you caught a cold. You call in sick and stay home the whole day covered up this time.

Scenario 17:

You are a tough kind of guy who does not listen to your parents. You always go out in the cold wearing just a t-shirt. Your parents have to practically force you before you wear a jacket or sweater. Then you catch a cold and now you are ready to listen and ask for help from your parents. You are willing to listen on how to treat a cold rather then how to prevent a cold. You realize that you don't know everything and that your parent's advice, no matter if you agree with it or not, is for your own good.

Scenario 18:

You are stranded somewhere cold and you have no food. You remember to find a place where you can spot help and conserve your energy by not moving too much. You also make sure to retain maximum body heat by using the technique and wearing layered clothes. Since the body does not need extra heat, it will burn less of the foods for heat. So whatever foods are left in your stomach will last you until your rescue arrives or until you spot help. You have gone two days without food, which is incredible. The survival training you received as a kid saved your life.

Chemical Temperature

Chinese people have known this fact for centuries about foods having some kind of temperature element to it. They incorporate it in their daily cooking. They have even developed many different mixtures of meats and vegetables to create an assortment of dishes which we call stir fry. A traditional Chinese meal usually comprises of meat and vegetable dishes so the temperature element in the dish is balanced. Chemical temperature is what the body produces by converting food and water into energy and heat. The chemical reaction in the food either heats you up and will raise blood pressure, or cool you down and lower blood pressure.

Scenario 19:

You are hungry but you are on a diet and refuse to eat anything that has fat. You have a salad without any meat. It fills up the emptiness in your stomach but a few hours later you start craving meat, but you still refuse to eat meat despite the body's request. You get tired very quickly and always need to munch on something to obtain energy.

The foods you eat don't give you long lasting energy. You finally give in and eat some meat and you can feel a burst of real energy throughout your body. Now you have energy to last the rest of the day.

Scenario 20:

You are like me, a meat lover. You must have some kind of meat in every meal you eat. You don't eat enough green so you start to get breakouts. You try all sorts of medications but the breakouts still occur. Then one day you decide to go on a diet so you eat a lot of salads and just a little meat for flavor. Within a week, your acne disappears and it does not return as long as you are on the diet plan. You stay on the diet for a month, and then you are back to your old self eating anything in sight, especially meats. You start developing acne again. You decided from that day on you would always try to eat a balanced meal which includes vegetables in your diet. The acne lessens to almost none.

Scenario 21:

It is the holiday and there are lots of foods, especially fried foods. You overeat because it tastes so good. The next day you start developing a mild cough and then it becomes worse the next couple of days. You tried to take all sorts of cough medications, cough syrups, and cough drops, and nothing seems to work. Your blood pressure is rising and you have no choice but to cut back on meat and eat salad for a week. Then you notice the cough gradually disappears without any use of medication.

Chap 6: Ying and yang

Everything we ingest, or shoot into the blood stream, or allow to absorb through the skin has a temperature element to it. The chemical reaction creates a heating or cooling effect. Chinese call this chemical reaction the **Ying and Yang** of foods because they believe in balancing their food intake. The ying is considered to be the heating aspect and it is most useful to keep the body warm and raise long lasting energy. The yang is considered to be the cooling aspect and useful to keep the ying in check and balanced. Notice how the symbol of the ying and yang is balance, they are both equally important. You can not have the ying over powering yang or the yang over powering ying.

There is a problem since 90% of all foods are ying and only 10% are yang, it is very hard to have a balanced meal. Meat and seafood are ying and even some fruits and vegetables are considered ying. That's not even including the difference type of nuts, drinks, and chemicals we ingest. How you prepare foods is also as important as what you prepare. Anything being fried or baked are considered being ying. If you fry a yang vegetable, it becomes ying as well. If your ying level is too high, in Chinese it is loosely translated as ***hot air***. So when I say you are full of hot air, I mean it literally. Only a few select items of food are really considered yang. When it comes to foods, the ying definitely dominates the yang and that is why it is so hard to stay in balance.

Luckily, there is a special cooling tea called chrysanthemum and it is made of chrysanthemum flower extract with sugar added. You need to brew real chrysanthemum flower if you want fresh ingredients and don't mind bitterness. This tea (yang) helps you balance the ying foods you eat everyday since a majority of us don't eat enough greens. It is convenient since you have to drink something along with your meal anyhow, why not drink chrysanthemum tea instead of your usual drink. It is recommenced that you drink it with room temperature water since the tea is meant to cool you down not heat you up or chill you.

There are those whose choice is to eat vegetables instead of drinking chrysanthemum tea to balance the ying foods. Vegetables have the shortest shelve life and are usually tasteless. It is the fat in meat that gives the vegetable taste. Chinese cooking usually cooks vegetables with meat because it is hard to just swallow plain vegetables. Unlike American cooking, the meat (flavorful) is separate from blanch or broiled vegetables (bland or tasteless), no wonder kids don't grow up liking vegetables. To make vegetables desirable and tasty, you must mix it up with meats and gravy so the taste is in balance and most important of all tasty.

Eating a balanced meal means you must include all of the food groups especially meat because it is the food of choice for long lasting energy. We are born with canine teeth for a reason and they are designed to eat meat. We have so many mixed messages about foods these days.

There is much debate on which foods are good for the body. Take the famous egg for example: we were told eggs are good for you one day and not the next. The public has to come to their own conclusion due to all the conflicting scientific reports. We never agree on anything and everyone has an opinion on everything especially what kinds of diets are healthy for the body. All diets are essentially unhealthy for the body because they are designed to starve the body and force the body to burn body fat for energy and heat. As long as the foods you eat are natural foods and you eat in moderation, it is good for the body. We can all agree that the body needs food to survive, then why are we restricting the body of it. Foods are what fuel and warm the body.

We are in a time where obesity is becoming a norm all over the world. With all these diets plans, America is still leading the world in obesity. We rush to blame meats for the obesity epidemic because it sounds right. The idea that by eating fat, you will get fat is wrong. To convince ourselves that eating fat is the cause of obesity, we have a fear of eating meat. *We should respect all foods not only some.* There are so many diet plans in existence today and none have really addressed the real cause of obesity until now. Now we even instill fear in eating carbohydrates because some scientists and doctors believe it is the real cause of obesity. As you walk down the grocery market aisle, all the signs either say low fat, fat free, light, or low in carbohydrates.

Before the low carb revolution, there was only a fear of fat in meat that caused obesity. Now we fear carbohydrates more than we fear the fat in meat. It is said that carbohydrates are easier to convert into sugar, which in turn becomes fat is also false. There is even a diet plan that promotes only eating meat over carbohydrates to loose weight. With all this contradicting health advice, how can you expect people to learn to stay healthy? All diet plans are extreme; they either abuse the body in terms of gluttony, poison, or by neglecting the body. We have experts from all walks of life dispensing nutritional advice and yet we are still no better off.

We are in a diet revolution created by society's image of what is beauty. Media opted to portray what they consider beautiful by sacrificing health to achieve it. The idea that being thin symbolizes health as well as beauty is false. Thin people deprive the body of nourishment, fat people over eat and abuse the body, and diets pills are poison for the body. None of these methods are the solution to obesity because it does not address the underling cause of obesity which is in the *drink* and not in the *foods or pills.* I will explain the answer to solving this epidemic in a later chapter.

Let's briefly discuss the many diets plan out there and the extreme methods people take to loose weight. There are the calorie count, low fat, low carbohydrate, diet pills, shakes, vegetarians, vomiting, and worse of all starvation diets.

The low fat diet was the most popular because dieters actually control and limit their own intake of fat. The fear was that the more fat you ate, the fatter you become. If that is true then why don't traditional Chinese people get fat eating greasy foods like Peking duck (one of many fattening foods). If you have ever eaten one, you know that 50% of the duck is nothing but fat. I ask a lot of people that question and their answer was that Chinese people eat a lot of rice and vegetables. That is true to a certain point but Chinese who adopt American diets still stay thin. So fat in foods is not the culprit in the obesity epidemic.

There are the calorie count (point) dieters. This diet limits the body's daily allowance of calories. Calorie numbers are set by so-called expert nutritionists, not the body. The notion that you can loose weight by controlling your calorie intake is absurd. Everyone has to become an expert nutritionist overnight just to be able to eat. Everything is labeled as though a few extra calories will affect your weight. The body is very resilient and can handle a lot more calories than we give it credit. You cannot go out to a restaurant because the menu doesn't have a nutritional label, so you can't make a sound decision.

The diet pills dieter are really poisoning the body. Dieters take pills to curb their appetite so they will not feel hungry. The body needs food to operate and instead the body receives pills which are artificial chemicals the body needs to eventually clean up. The pills numb the hungry feeling so the body is forced to seek alternative fuel which happens to be the body's fat. Prolonged use of these diets will result in a weak body as the body will start burning muscle tissue and organs once it depletes its body fat resources.

The shakes dieter uses a diet known as a liquid lunch diet. This diet replaces traditional meals with shakes or smoothies because it is already in liquid form so it is effortless for the body to process and convert into energy and heat. The nutritional value in the drink will sustain you and provide you with energy for the day. Just think of this diet as a multi-vitamin regimen in liquid form. These diets can cost you lots of money. ***My motto is, "if you need to eat to survive, why not enjoy it?"*** The liquid lunch lacks a lot of nutrients only found in natural foods.

The low carbohydrate diet is the most recent diet out there. The theory is that carbohydrates converts easily into glucose and is absorbed by the body. By reducing the carbohydrate intake, the body will not have that much carbohydrate to convert into fat. The fear of eating white rice is instilled in the public's mind because of the carbs. If that is true then why are Chinese people eating so many carbohydrates (white rice) everyday not obese like Americans?

A vegetarians' diet consists of only vegetables and no meats. Some believe this diet will help them slim down and stay thin. The body is forced to burn excess (body) fat since you deprive the body of the nutrient (fat) it needs. Vegetarians are thin but they are very unhealthy because the body's yang is over powered by ying. The body is weak and vulnerable to developing disease without a real source of fuel (meat).

There is the vomiting diet (bulimia) which is very serious and deadly. You eat all the delicious foods you desire and then you vomit it out so the foods won't stay in your body long enough to turn into fat. This form of diet neglects the body's need for nutrients and when the body runs out of reserve (excess) fat to burn, the body is forced to rob nutrients from the muscles, organs, and/or bones. This is a serious matter that can lead to death.

The last type of diets is a starvation diet (anorexia) where a person does not eat at all (fast) for days or weeks. Water is the only thing they live on. These ultimate diets can kill because the body cannot survive long without food. It is the most severe diets of them all. Even the vomiting diet is not as bad as these diets. At least in the vomiting diet, there are still some foods left in the body.

Scenario 22:

Like many Americans, you too don't bring lunch to work. You eat out mostly fast foods because of the lunch time restriction. Your meal is definitely not balanced. The foods are greasy and have little or no green vegetables. Your ying level is up to the roof and you get a heavy feeling for the rest of the day. When you got home, all you ate was a big bowl of salad and hardly any meat so it helped to raise the yang level. By balancing ying lunch you have at work, you feel much better and the heavy feeling subsides.

Scenario 23:

You are a big beer drinker and you got a big beer belly to prove it. Drinking beer to you is like drinking water. You need to drink more and more beers just to get the buzz you used to get when you first started drinking. Your body is beginning to be numb and you need to step up to hard liquor so you can get a buzz quicker. To you hard liquor has less carbohydrates and calories than beer so you don't gain more weight. When you discover your liver and kidneys are failing you due to drinking, you quit drinking and allow the body a chance to repair what is left of your liver and kidneys.

Scenario 24:

You are a vegetarian and refuse to eat meat for fear of fat, and you also respect animals too much to eat them. You always lack energy and catch colds easily. Your yang level is too low and you need to take a lot of vitamins to replace the nutrition you deprived the body of. You watch as your health condition worsens year after year. You are a prime candidate to develop a chronic disease because your body stays cold like a corpse. You heard from a friend that to regain your health you must start eating meat. So you try eating meat and your health keeps getting better and better.

Foods may have a ying or yang element in them but the body may have some difficulty processing certain foods depending on its composition or mixture. Once the foods are mixed up inside your stomach, you run the problem of **food interaction.** The foods itself may be safe but combined with certain other foods can create an adverse reaction known as allergies. Some people are allergic to certain foods because their bodies have not built up tolerance (immunity) for it yet. These foods can be safe for most but for a few it can be lethal.

Many of us suffer from malnutrition and need to take supplements just to function for the day. People who take **supplements** are wasting money and get fewer benefits than people who take natural foods. Yes supplements have ying and yang elements. *Why take supplements when you can take the real thing?* Supplements never have as much health and nutritional benefits as real foods do. It's a fact that over cooking vegetables depletes most of the vital nutrients found in a vegetable. I am sure that cooked vegetables still have more nutrients than vitamins do. Remember vitamins are chemically designed as a substitute for real natural foods.

Beside food, the body also needs **water** to survive. You can just live off water for days. Water is essential for digestion and hydrating the body but most American drinks are made with too many man-made chemicals. The chemical drinks such as soda, alcohol, or drink mix become a health risk. Man-made chemicals are toxic and have little or no nutritional value. The body only needs the water content to survive not all the other chemicals added. The body eventually needs to filter the chemicals out of the system through the kidneys. Water itself is the cleanest drink for the body and the more you add to the drink the unhealthier it becomes.

Alcohol is the worse drink of them all because it is nothing but poison for the body. Alcohol is made up of rotten fruit. Once you ferment the fruit and age it, the drink becomes toxic. Can you imagine leaving fruit to rot in its purest form and then eating it? That's what you are essentially doing. Notice the longer you allow the alcohol to age the stronger it becomes. Every time you drink alcohol, your heart beats extra hard to create more blood so it can clear out the toxin. That's why people drink alcohol to stay warm, but they are putting lots of stress on the heart. There are reports that say a glass of red wine a day along with your dinner is good for the heart. If that it is true then why can't children drink it for their heart? Alcohol is either a healthy drink or a poisonous drink for the body. There are no in-betweens where it is good for some and bad for others. When it comes to the body, a drink is either nutritious or poisonous.

People who drink coffee in the morning run on caffeine (artificial fuel) and when it wears off you get withdrawals and need to drink another cup just to have energy to last through the day. The non-coffee drinker runs on natural foods which is the purest form of fuel for the body and there are no withdrawal symptoms. Coffee drinkers are increasing by the millions and even teenager are getting hook on this addictive drink. Coffee is like a drug but people don't treat it like one. We all know that it is bad for us, but yet a majority of us rely on it for a temporary boost of energy in the morning.

Don't forget the most popular drink of them all, soda. People are drinking soda with their meal for the water requirement but depositing a lot of harmful chemicals into the body in the process. Instead of drinking plain water (tasteless), we are brain washed by the media to drink soda and artificial drinks full of lethal chemicals. The acid in the soda in high concentrations can burn a hole in the stomach. Notice when you pour a soda onto the ground and it fizzles. Those fizzles are the artificial acid in the soda. It is unhealthy to drink so many lethal chemicals. That does not mean you ban it all together. You can occasionally have soda as a treat because your body will have the time to clean out the toxins.

Scenario 25:

It is the final semester and you don't have any more time to waste because the test is tomorrow. You must study for the final and you become hungry. Instead of taking some time to go out and eat, you opted to drink lots of coffee to stay awake. You got through finals and when you got home you are very hungry. You start cleaning out the refrigerator by devouring anything that isn't nailed down. You feel very sleepy after eating and slept for the rest of the day.

Scenario 26:

You have a thin figure like a supermodel and you are a vegetarian with a fear of eating fat. You lack some nutrients in your diet, mainly protein, so you take vitamins as a replacement for meat. You got sick one day and had no energy at all despite your increased vitamin intake. You are constantly cold and can't seem to stay warm. Your health got worse until you started eating a balanced meal which included meat. You notice your energy level increasing and you gradually feel better.

Scenario 27:

Everywhere you go, your choice of drink is plain water. When the water selection was out in the vending machine, you would rather stay thirsty than drink a soda. Then one day during a sports game, you were thirsty and wanted to buy bottled water, unfortunately, they were sold out. Your alternative was juice and they were sold out too. You stay thirsty while you watch your friends and the audience enjoying their sodas. The game is a couple of hours away from ending and you can't wait that long, so you finally decided to purchase a soda to quench your thirst. Breaking the vow you made to yourself lifted a ton of weight off your mind.

Air Temperature

It is well documented that humans in general are shallow breathers. We only use a small portion of our lung capacity. We live in a hectic time when breathing is not a priority. Many times I have told people to breathe because they were complaining of being tired. Their response was I am breathing or else I would die. Subconsciously, your mind will help you breathe the minimum (not enough) to be healthy, so the body becomes tired. It is the body's way of warning you that it lacks oxygen. *Is there one thing in this world that is truly free which we are not utilizing?* The answer is the air we breathe. People have owned everything else but the air itself. It is free to those who value and reap its rewards. Oxygen is a necessity just like food and water. We tie up the mind with so much junk and tend to forget to make it a priority to breathe. You are no good to others if you don't take care of yourself and are healthy.

Scenario 28:

You have one of those boring jobs where you just sit and day dream. There is nothing to do but you somehow feel tired for some reason. You try to figure out what is causing you to be tired all the time. It couldn't be lack of sleep because you devoted a full eight hours of sleep just as recommended by doctors. It also couldn't be food related because you just ate breakfast. Then you suddenly figure out that breathing is the only thing you keep forgetting to do. You were so busy thinking about daily chores that breathing properly takes the back seat. Now that you know the cause of your constant tiredness, you start taking five minute breathing breaks when ever you feel tired.

Scenario 29:

It is Christmas time in retail and you are so busy that you don't even have time to eat less remember to breathe. Customers have you running around like a chicken with its' head cut off. Your mind is rushing to help multiple customers at one time. This multitasking stress burns you out. You finally have a chance to take your lunch. After lunch, you are still somehow feeling tired. Then a co-worker reminds you to breathe so you start breathing as you help customers. Your energy returns quickly and for the rest of the day you have a smile on your face rather than a frown.

Scenario 30:

Everything is not going according to plan. Your mind is stuck on solving a particular problem. You start to get very tired and really need energy boost. You ate a lot but your energy level doesn't seem to rise as fast as you would like. You drink more water hoping that will solve your lack of energy, and it helps a little. You remember what your dad has taught you before that breathing helps you get your energy back. You were amazed at the results after a few minutes of breathing exercises. Every break from then on is a breathing break.

Chap 7: Breathing technique

There is regular breathing and a special technique to breathing. When you move and use lots of strength, your body needs oxygen and food for energy. When you don't breathe enough oxygen, you will start to get tired and sweat. The body can not really speak and let you know what is wrong, but it can display symptoms to warn you it is being abused or neglected. Oxygen is cooling in nature while carbon dioxide is heating in nature. Do this experiment to prove it to yourself. Stand close to a mirror and just blow at it and you will realize that you are blowing oxygen (cool) and not carbon dioxide (hot). Now simulate the fogging of the mirror with your breathe, you will realize that it is the carbon dioxide (hot) air that is coming out not the oxygen (cool).

This is a breathing technique I came up with and it is very similar to the slow breathing technique. You start inhaling minimally through the nose and fogging out maximally through the mouth. Do it for five minutes if you are feeling tired, then you will regain your energy and stop sweating. I know you were taught to inhale through the nose as much as you exhale through your mouth. This breathing technique is old and does not work as well.

Let's use a bottle to represent the lungs, clean water represents oxygen, and dirty water represents carbon dioxide. Let's for sake of argument fill the bottle full of dirty water (lungs full of carbon dioxide) and try to replace the dirty water in the bottle with fresh water (replace carbon dioxide in lungs with oxygen). You can't pour any fresh water in since the bottle (lungs) is already filled with dirty water (you cannot inhale because the lungs are already full of carbon dioxide). **The law of space states that no two things (oxygen & carbon dioxide) can occupy the same space.**

Let's examine the old technique and pretend the bottle is half filled with dirty water (lung is half full of carbon dioxide). You pour the fresh water in (inhale) and before the fresh water reaches the dirty water (the oxygen reaches your lungs), you pour out the fresh water you just poured in (exhale the fresh air you just inhaled). That's why when you exhale, the air is cool (oxygen) not hot (carbon dioxide). You are essentially back to square one. Even though you manage to pour out some dirty water (exhale small portions of the carbon dioxide), you need to find a lot of time to do breathing exercises such as yoga and meditation. Let's now examine Pei's breathing technique and pretend 90% of the bottle is filled with dirty water (90% of lungs full of carbon dioxide). Pour in as little as possible fresh water (inhale for a minimum of one second) and then pour out as much of the dirty water as possible (fog out as long as you have breath). Notice by pouring out all the dirty water (fogging out hot air not blowing out cool air), the bottle (lungs) is empty to carry all the fresh water you want (room to inhale as much oxygen you desire). Do this simple experiment to prove it to yourself. It is a simple technique but very effective. Now you do not have any excuse not to breathe properly. I know you have a couple of minutes to spare. You can do this breathing technique anytime and anywhere.

As you do the breathing technique, your lungs will began filling up with fresh air. The blood around the lungs receives all the oxygen it needs while the rest of the body is deprived because you are sitting still. You need to get up and walk or move around so the blood will circulate. Eventually the oxygenated blood will replace the oxygen depleted blood. Tiredness is simply the body's way of letting you know that the blood lacks oxygen. If you don't give the body what it needs, you will experience not only tiredness but asthma like symptoms or shortness of breath.

I too used to have shortness of breath from time to time. The first time it happened, I panicked like every one else and catching a deep breathe was the only thing on my mind. The harder I tried to take a deep breathe, the more tense and agitated I became. I thought I was developing asthma. Ever since I discovered the breathing technique, I was very excited. At first, I thought it was just a fluke and it would not work every time. I guess I was wrong because it works every single time I or anyone else uses the technique. Now I incorporate the breathing technique in everything I do.

Smokers of course will develop problem breathing because every cigarette you smoke will reduce the capacity of your lungs to carry oxygen. It is bad enough we have to subject the lungs to air pollution, but we also volunteer to infect it with cigarette smoke as well. There are so many health problems related to smoking. Even the cigarette box has the surgeon general's warning on it forewarning us of the potential risk. Not to mention second hand smoke and the unborn. There are countless ads paid for by Cigarette

Companies to educate the public about the danger of cigarettes and information on how one can quit smoking. Why should you start something you eventually have to quit either voluntarily or by force from your doctor or loved one? Remember you only get compliments and praise one time when you smoke your first cigarette. After that you are just stuck living with a nasty addiction. I guess it is true that bad habits die hard. Because the cigarette has lots of harmful chemicals, the heart needs to raise the blood pressure to clean up the toxins. Most smokers die of heart complications, then cancer of the lungs due to cigarette smoke. When the body raises its blood pressure to clean out the toxins, the body converts more foods into heat. That means if your ying is not balanced, you will get sick with cold, fever, flu, headache, cough, etc.

Air Particles

Every year we contribute to the pollution of the air. We breathe in all these pollutants we call air particles. Air particles we breathe in every day include dust, allergens, pollen, carbon monoxide, etc. It can create a lot of breathing problems like asthma and allergies in some people. Air particles can also include germs, bacteria, or viruses which can make you very sick. The air particles first enter the body through the nose as we breathe. The nose hair is the body's first line of defense by trapping the air particles. If there are too many particles to inhale, the body will cause you to sneeze and out come the particles. If that is not enough, the body creates mucus to trap the particles so minimal particles enter your body. A runny nose is a way the body clears the debris trapped in the nose. How severe particles effect people is determined by the person's own ying level.

The higher the ying level, the more sensitive you are to particles. Especially be careful of viruses because it tends to lodge itself in the throat causing you a lot of misery. The particles can trigger the body's defense mechanism which means the body needs to raise it's temperature and if the ying and yang are not balanced then the body will warn you by displaying symptoms.

Scenario 31:

You just ate at home and you feel sleepy and you don't know why. Luckily you have nothing planned for the afternoon so you took a nap and woke up feeling refreshed. The next day while at work you feel sleepy again after lunch but you can't just take a nap like you normally do when your home. So you try washing your face with cold water which helps a little. You start the breathing technique and that makes you even sleepier. You got up and walked outside to get fresh air while you continued practicing the breathing technique. Your energy quickly returns and you stop feeling sleepy. The combination of the breathing technique and moving around is the key for you to regain your energy.

Scenario 32:

You are otherwise in good health but now and then you can't seem to catch your breathe. Doctors say you might have a mild case of asthma but you refuse to accept it. The asthma like symptoms comes and goes so you just live with it. Your life is very stressful with so many things on your mind at every waking moment. You took some meditation classes that help you with your breathing. Whenever you have too much on your mind, you will always make time to practice the breathing technique.

Scenario 33:

You have been smoking for forty long years and your lungs are about to give out on you. You are limited down to three choices: you can quit smoking voluntarily or forced, and allow the body time to recover, obtain transplanted lungs and live hooked up to a respirator, or just wait for death. You don't want to die so soon because you want to live to see your grandchildren. Yes the joy of being a grandparent, you have all the benefits of spoiling your grandchildren without the responsibility of raising them. You don't have the time or the money to wait for transplants. You don't want to live hooked up to a respirator because it limits your mobility and is very expensive to maintain. Your only option left is to volunteer to quit smoking because you don't want the doctors or your loved ones to force you. They will make you quit cold turkey.

Absorption rate

Absorption rate is the percentage of processible foods divided by the percentage of waste in the body. The stomach only has a limited amount of space to carry either foods or waste. Since the food and waste cannot occupy the same space, if your meal is one pound heavy and you only relieve half a pound, where is the other half of the meal? It doesn't just magically disappear. As the percentage of processible foods increases, the percentage of body waste decreases, and the higher the absorption rate is. As the percentage of processible foods decreases, the percentage of body waste increases, and the lower the absorption rate is. For example, you have a delicious apple and you want the body to absorb 100% of the nutrient from the apple. You eat the apple and it goes into the digestive track to be processed and converted into energy and heat, but you have twice the amount of waste in your stomach. The nutritious apple is mixed with the waste and the body cannot absorb 100% of the apple. The solution is to flush out the waste first. Then when you eat the apple, there will only be the apple in the digestive track, so 100% absorption rate is possible. The real reason why some people gain weight while others do not is based solely on the body's absorption rate.

Doctors and nutritionists all agree about the three major contributing factors that cause the development of body fat. They are the sugar, fat, and carbohydrates in foods. It is time to demystify the fear of the dreadful three that experts claim to cause the obesity epidemic in America. Sugar, fat, and carbohydrates are healthy and natural nutrients for the body in moderation. How could something so good as well as a necessity for the body be feared rather than appreciated? The dreadful three are among the many nutrients which the body needs to operate on. Every diet known to man consists of controlling the intake of one or more of the dreadful three.

It is during this century that obesity has risen rapidly. What has changed to cause this phenomenon? The doctors and nutritionists with all their expertise in diets plan have all fail to solve a simple problem. They ask the wrong questions so they all get the wrong answers. The question is not what is in the food that causes weight gain. The right question to ask is at what temperature we should consume our drinks. Food itself does not harm the body, the way we treat food does.

Scenario 34:

You have always been a health conscious person. You watch what you eat and count every calorie. You monitored your intake of sugar because you were told by many experts that eating over your daily allowance of sugar will cause you to gain weight. Of course the fear they instill in you carries into adulthood, and many times you control you're craving so you won't jeopardize your diet. You attend parties but never really enjoy yourself because you nickel and dime every food you eat that has dreaded three. The foods at the party don't have labels with their nutritional value so you opt to not eat most of the time. The only foods that are safe to eat are mostly vegetables.

Scenario 35:

You love to eat meats of all sorts. It was a dream come true when you heard that there was a diet plan that teaches you to only eat meat and vegetables to loose weight. You quickly purchased the book and started the new diet plan. Your weight comes off but your blood pressure is through the roof, but you don't really care as long as you loose the weight. There is only one thing you don't really like about this diet and that is you have to stop eating practically all foods that have carbohydrates in them. This means you have to give up your favorite foods like pizza, hamburger, and hot dogs.

Scenario 36:

You are the traditional dieter who looks for anything labeled low fat or fat free. The fat content on the label is very important to you. You will not eat anything that has fat that is over the limit you have set for yourself to follow. During picnics, instead of eating barbecue ribs like everyone else, you brought your own foods that have hardly any fat in them. Everyone looked at you thinking you hate the foods they have prepared. You have to explain your diet restriction every time you attend a function or gathering.

Everyone seems happy and smiling except you, maybe because you feel like you do not fit in.

Chap 8: Waste

Waste are merely foods that are depleted of it nutrients and need to be discarded from the body. If left in the body too long, waste becomes toxic to the body. Could you imagine foods from a week ago still stuck rotting in the stomach? The toxic waste causes many diseases and discomfort in people. Waste takes up unnecessary space in the stomach as well. It stretches the stomach lining so the stomach needs to make room to carry foods. Waste is also dead weight which you need a lot of energy to lug around. The more waste in the stomach, the more processible foods you need because your absorption rate is decreasing. If foods are frozen in the stomach, they are also considered to be waste. Because the body is unable to process the frozen foods it might as well be waste.

Let us use the famous American greasy meal of a hamburger, fries, and a cold drink to illustrate the difference between American ways of eating versus Chinese eating techniques. We will have Joe eat the same meal, and just to be fair the only things we will change is the type of beverage Joe drinks. Every person I shared this information with stated, "I never thought about it like that but you are right." You will say that too after you learn the real reason why hardly any Chinese people get fat.

Cold drinks

Ever since the invention of the refrigerator, Americans exploit the real reason it was made for. The purpose of the refrigerator is to store foods so it will last longer, not to keep the drinks chilled. Life in America has become more and more hectic as both parents need to work to make a living, so there is little time left to shop for foods. Buying in bulk to save a buck or two is becoming very common in every household. Some foods are even eaten cold instead of hot such as salads with dressing and sandwiches (cold cuts). The food and drink industries have created a dependency on cold drinks and foods so much that every restaurant and fast food chain conveniently serves their foods and drinks cold. We have grown so accustomed to cold drinks that we won't drink if it isn't chilled. Could you drink room temperature soda or water? The majority of us can't, that is why weight gain has become such a big issue. Ice becomes a necessity in all drinks because drinks are not left in the refrigerator long enough to be chilled. Even alcoholic drinks which are meant to keep the body warm by raising blood pressure are on the rocks (ice) these days. Juices of all sorts are kept chilled in the fridge. Milk is chilled and so is water. Beers are served cold and especially sodas. American's favorite beverages are chilled or it won't taste good. Every single beverage American's drink is chilled; no wonder there is an obesity crisis in America. Tea which is traditionally served hot is turned into ice tea. The fridge even dispenses ice. When did the refrigerator change from just storing foods to being an ice maker as well? The stomach is always kept cool so foods get stuck in the small intestine too long and the body will store the fat away for emergency use. This is what John used to tell me. ***You can't burn fat in a cold oven (stomach or torso).*** If you treat the body like a refrigerator, how do you expect the body to burn anything? You voluntarily create internal temperature chaos which is worse because you are causing it not the ambient temperature.

We will start with the American diet first. We will use Joe as a subject in both scenarios. As Joe takes a bite of the food and the grease coats his esophagus, Joe chases it down with a big gulp of the chilled soda. The cold temperature of the soda congeals and coagulates the oil in his esophagus causing the grease to be stuck there. Joe has the same meal as lunch five times a week because his work restricts him from eating a balanced meal. Since Joe keeps the oil frozen in the esophagus, the body has to build up stomach acid to reach and melt the oil down. Joe has acid reflux disease and needs to pop an acid reducer after every meal. The stomach acid level is too high and is eating away at the stomach lining and creating an ulcer. Joe also gets a heavy feeling after every meal even though Joe tries to eat a lot of vegetables at home. The diet at home doesn't help because he still consumes cold drinks at home. The purpose of a drink along with a meal is to help the body flush the foods throughout the body. The body is only interested in the water content not all the other chemicals added to the drink. The cold drink keeps the foods frozen in Joe's stomach for days. Joe has a hard time going to the restroom because he is always constipated. The waste is building up in Joe's stomach. Every time Joe uses the restroom, it is very painful because his stools are very hard and large. His stool tears his anus, causing him to have hemorrhoids. His anus bleeds easily. Joe's stomach becomes larger and he needs to eat more and more to get the same energy he used to get to function for the day. The waste in his stomach prevents the body from relaxing so he cannot get a good night's rest. When Joe wakes up in the morning, he has no energy and needs coffee to give him an artificial boost of energy that lasts a couple of hours.

Let's do an experiment to prove it to yourself. Take a cup and fill it with cooking oil and then pour it out to simulate the esophagus coated with oil. Now try to get rid of the oil by flushing it with cold water and watch how the oil congeals or coagulates by sticking to the cup. Now use room temperature water to clean the oil and then feel the cup with your fingers and you will see that the oil still remains stuck in the cup. That is what really happens in the stomach. You may argue that the body can warm up the water and foods you eat. However, do you know how much heat it takes to warm up icy water, or how long it takes to warm up room temperature water? It takes a lot of processible foods to produce such heat. When you want to boil water do you use the hot water from the tap, room temperature water, or cold water? Why? The answer is simple, the hotter the water already is the less energy you need to boil the water. The colder the water is, the more energy you need to boil the water.

I still remember when I was younger, I used to drink everything cold no matter if it was winter time or summer time. My mom would cringe whenever she saw me chill my drink. I did not know any better so I too have gone through all the symptoms and suffering brought on by cold drinks. Every winter time, I would develop a nasty cough that I could not seem to shake. It would lessen one day and come right back in full force the next, and sometimes worse than before. I always thought that I had some sort of allergy that only surfaced during certain times of the year. I would never figure it was because I kept the body cold all the time by drinking cold drinks. Now I understand why; I was not adequately keeping my body warm so temperature chaos affected my body from outside as well as inside.

Scenario 37:

You drink soda your whole life and can't give it up. You must drink at least two cans of soda with every meal and it must be chilled. Your sodas of choice are colas and you need it for energy to function. You need the sugar fix because the foods are frozen by the soda in your stomach. You are running on caffeine and sugar which wears off very quickly. You have a hard time going to sleep because the body is constantly kept cold. When you wake up, you feel exhausted and need a lot of caffeine and sugar to stay awake. You also eat very little meat products so you always complain of being tired and don't know why.

Scenario 38:

You are not into sodas but you drink room temperature water because you were told by doctors to flush your system with water. You hardly eat any meat because the fat goes directly to your stomach, hips, and thighs. You drink plenty of water every day but yet you always lack energy and need to constantly munch on something. You spread your meal into small portions so that your body can have time to digest the foods. You don't refrigerate your water because it is too cold for you to drink. The oil is still stuck in your esophagus so you get acid reflux once in a while, but you don't really care because it is not serious.

Scenario 39:

You eat anything that is tasty and usually overeat in most cases and drink very little water. Whenever you feel tension and discomfort due to the body feeling cold, you take a shot of whiskey and feel warmth all over your body. Alcohol elevates your heart to beat at an incredible rate. Your tension temporarily numbed for the moment and you no longer feel cold. You have a glass of red wine with your meal because your doctor says it is good for the heart. It seems that alcohol is your choice of drink on the dinner table.

Hot drinks

Before the invention of the refrigerator, only one parent needed to work to support the family so the stay at home parent had time to go grocery shopping. There is always one parent at home cooking, usually the wife or mother. Since there were no means of storing foods and keeping beverages chilled, traditional Chinese families were accustomed to drinking hot drinks, especially hot tea. Their meals are always consisting of hot food, hot tea and/or hot soup. There is a saying the Chinese always use, "eat while it is still piping hot." Chinese foods and drinks are hot in nature while the opposite is true about American foods and drinks. If you ever go to an authentic Chinese restaurant, you will notice that they serve you hot tea before you even order. Hot soups are always eaten as an appetizer, and after the meal the desert is served hot as well as sweet. Remember that hot soup works as well as any hot drink to get rid of the oil buildup in the body. Have you ever wondered why they serve tea in such a small cup instead of a large supersized cup that Americans are accustomed to drinking? It is a custom and a secret which I am going to share with you. The reason why Chinese restaurants serve tea in such a small cup is because they want you to drink the hot tea along with your meal, not only after your meal. If the cup is too large, it will take too long for the tea to cool down enough for you to drink without burning yourself. The cups are designed small because by the time you have eaten a bite or two of the food, the hot tea will cool down enough for you to drink. You have essentially created a sandwich effect where the hot tea is sandwiched in between the many layers of foods. The layer of hot tea helps soften the many layered foods so the body can process the foods into energy and body heat easier. The essential oil in tea leaf is shown to break down oil. Hot water alone is good to break down oil, but hot tea (hot water with detergent) is even better.

Now Joe will eat the same meal except the drink will be hot tea rather than his usual cold drink. As Joe takes a bite of the hamburger, the oil coats his esophagus. He sips some hot tea and can feel the heat in the esophagus and stomach area. The hot tea breaks down and flushes the oil out of Joe's system. Joe no longer gets the greasy and heavy feeling he normally gets eating burgers and fries. The hot tea also helps Joe by softening the waste so the journey through his small intestine is effortless. He also rid himself of acid reflux disease. When he goes to relieve himself, foods from yesterday come out smoothly and Joe does not have a hemorrhoid problem any longer. Joe's absorption rate increases as he adopts the new technique of eating foods. The hot tea got rid of the waste and helped the body digest foods more efficiently. The fat and sugar are not left in the body long enough for it to become a problem.

The body absorbs all the nutrients it needs and the rest are flushed out by the hot tea.

If you ever wash dishes, you will know what I mean. Only hot temperature water can break down and remove the oil molecules from dishes. Hot water alone can clean the oil but hot water with detergent (tea) is even better at cleaning the oil. The answer to the obesity problem is quite simple, but no one ever thought like this before that is why it has eluded experts. It makes perfect sense that it takes heat to burn fat but as long as people treat the body like a refrigerator rather than an oven, we will always be stuck with this problem. No diet plan has ever addressed the issue of heat in drinks as the real cause of obesity. We must stop focusing our attention on what is in the foods and focus more on the temperature of the drink. *It is not what you eat that makes you fat but how you eat it.*

Scenario 40:

You don't eat out a lot so you can save money. Therefore, you always bring your own lunch to work. This way you can always include your bowl of hot soup with your lunch. When you do go out for a special occasion, you choose to go to a Chinese restaurant because they serve hot soup and hot tea. You do not have acid reflux disease like many of your friends who only eat American dishes. No matter what you eat or drink during the day, you always make sure you drink a cup of hot tea or hot water before bed.

Scenario 41:

For some reason you love eating Chinese foods even though you are not Chinese. Maybe because you don't get the usual heartburn, indigestion, and bloating you get from eating anywhere else. You even learn to use chopsticks to eat instead of a fork and spoon. You are a regular at a particular Chinese restaurant where they call you by your name. You love the hot tea and hot soup they serve you. You usually eat alone because most of your friends don't share your taste for Chinese foods like you do. You too don't really care for the soul foods which they happen to like eating everyday.

Scenario 42:

You love eating a bowl of hot noodle soup because it is easy to swallow. If you are eating rice and there is hot soup, you would combine the two to make rice soup. Everyone in your family looks at you strangely as though you have committed a crime or something. You like it because you don't need to eat a lot of other dishes of foods. There is always extra soup made because they know how much you like to drink soup. Even in the summer when you are eating out, your first choice is a bowl of hot noodle soup any time of the day.

Rest

We tend to take rest for granted because it takes up too much of our precious waking hour's time. We always test the limitation of the body by depriving the body of rest time it deserves. We opted to stay up late and wake up early so we have more waking hours time to do things. We put so much demand on the body to perform at top condition, but we do not allow it enough rest. The body uses rest as a time to recover itself from daily activities. Sooner or later the sleep deprived body will catch up to you and you will have no choice but to just collapse, giving the body much needed rest. The body cannot shut down completely or else you will die, so it goes into the idle mode similar to a car idling in park. The body still needs food for energy and heat so it can repair itself of any abuse or neglect imposed on the body during the day. No matter what treatments you may seek from any doctor, they all recommend one thing and that is plenty of rest. It is because of rest that the body can ever get well.

Time

During rest, the body needs a certain amount of time to repair itself depending on the severity of the problem. *It is not the quantity of sleep that the body needs but the quality of sleep.* It is said that the couple of hours before waking up is when the body goes into deep sleep. However, based on Pei System, you can help the body enter into deep sleep the very first hour in bed. This means you do not need a lot of hours of sleep and the body still gets enough rest. The recommendation of eight hours of sleep for adults is outdated and is now being revised. We do not determine the amount of sleep the body needs, the body will let you know if it is lacks sleep or not. It is said that we spend one third of our lives sleeping, why not make every hour count?

In order to help the body to enter deep sleep during the first hour, the body must meet four necessary criteria:

- First of all, you must feed the body foods so the body won't go hungry, especially some meat for energy to last through the long night.
- Secondly, help the body achieve and maintain equilibrium by applying the pillow technique so the body can relax itself.

- Thirdly, you must oxygenate the blood by using the breathing technique.
- Finally, you must relax the mind or else you will never go to sleep. ***The body is awake if the mind is awake.***

If any of the four criteria are not met, the body will take longer to go into deep sleep. Before you wake up in the morning, you will feel energized but for some reason you do not want to get out of bed. Open your eyes so it helps to wake the mind up. Take fifteen minutes to practice the breathing technique. It will get rid of that weird feeling of not wanting to get up because the body is too comfortable in bed. It is natural since the body is lacking just a little more oxygen in the blood to transition from sleeping mode to waking mode.

Digestion

Digestion is a major issue when we talk about weight gain. How well the body digests foods will determine the level of metabolism in a person. It is blamed on genetics for those who cannot lose weight due to a low metabolism. The body does not store fat just because doctors say you inherit a fat gene. Based on the Pei System, it is the mistreatment of foods that causes the body to store fat, not the content of the foods or whether you are genetically programmed to be fat. What do you expect the body to do when you leave frozen foods in the stomach for days by drinking cold drinks? Once the blood absorbs all the nutrients it needs, then the body assumes you want to store away the rest of the frozen foods for emergency use, which is why you don't get rid of it right away. The term metabolizes means to burn not store fat.

A healthy person has regularity every single day. Regularities are important because it tells you that any unused foods left in the stomach are being disposed of in a timely manner. Today's foods should be out of the system the next day, not a couple days later. Foods which are nourishing to the body turns into toxic waste if left in the body too long. Millions of Americans are constantly constipated and don't know why. Their digestion is very poor so the foods are not properly processed into energy and heat. Have you ever heard the phrase "catch 22?" In this situation, the body needs the energy from the frozen foods in the stomach in order to convert itself (frozen foods) into energy and heat. In other words, the body does not have the necessary source of energy to process foods because the very source of energy is frozen within the foods; which the body needs to process into energy and heat. Will only drinking hot drinks instead of cold drinks solve these problems? Hot drinks will help the body heat up the foods rather than freezing it so the body can process the foods into energy and heat easier.

Let's see if I can explain it by using an example: We all know that gasoline to power a car is derived from crude oil. Imagine that there is a special car (body) that can convert crude oil (food) into gas (nutrients) but the car (body) needs gas (nutrients) to process the crude oil (food). What if you encase the crude oil (freeze the foods) and allow only a small portion (processible foods) to be processed (turned into nutrients). Where will the car (body) find enough gas (nutrients) to convert (turns) crude oil (foods) into more gas (nutrients)?

Scenario 43:

It is a long drive home and you did not get enough sleep before you headed out. You have to work the next day so you have no time to lose. You nodded off several times and nearly caused an accident. You stop at a rest stop and use the public restroom to wash your face with cold water hoping that will wake you up. You stay awake the next hour and then you feel sleepy again. You stop for a cup of coffee and that helps you a little and you get through another hour of driving. You finally decide to stop at the next rest stop and just take a quick nap. You nap for an hour and you wake up feeling refreshed and energized to drive the rest of the way. You learn your lesson from that experience that there is no substitute for rest.

Scenario 44:

You have a nasty cough that lasts for months and it seems to never go away. You take all sorts of drugs, tried all sort of remedies, and you are constantly taking cough drops to suppress it, but the cold still there. The cough gets worse as the weather gets colder. You can feel a lot of pain in your chest every time you cough. Luckily, a friend of yours tells you that eating a lot of green vegetables helps with a cough. You are so desperate that you would try anything despite your skepticism. You have nothing but salad for two days straight and the cough slowly subsides. You discover that there are no magic pills and it takes time for the body to correct and heal itself.

Scenario 45:

You have the traditional American meal everyday. Your digestion of foods is very poor and you feel sluggish and constipated all the time. You develop an ulcer and your doctor prescribes more pills for you. The condition never goes away until a friend gets you hooked on eating Chinese foods. You change from drinking cold drinks with your meal to drinking hot tea. After a week of eating Chinese food and drinking hot tea, you notice that your ulcer is not as severe and you feel more energy then ever before. You stop drinking cold drinks from that day on.

Blood circulation

Without blood, there will be no life as we speak. The purpose of the Pei System is solely to aid the blood by feeding it, oxygenating it, and helping it to avoid temperature chaos and achieve and maintain equilibrium by using the RS and Pillow Techniques. In order to replenish and oxygenate the blood at the extremities, the blood needs to constantly circulate itself, even during sleep. The blood should flow smoothly without any interference from internal or external temperature chaos caused by ambient temperature or cold drinks.

Chap 10: Exercise

We all agree that exercise is good for the body, but excessive exercise is bad, especially for the heart. Some exercise to stay in shape and strengthen the heart muscles while others exercise as a means to loose weight. We are led to believe by doctors that lack of exercise is what contributes to obesity in youth. Exercise is one of the reasons but not the only one. It is a combination of abuse and/or neglect on our part that causes obesity. Every time you exercise, the heart pumps blood extra hard and if the heart is pushed to its limits, then you stand a chance it might give out on you. Exercise is merely one of many ways to trigger the heart to work over time (raising body temperature above the equilibrium). External and internal temperature chaos can elevate heart rates and so will drugs and alcohol. Digestion problems and waste can trigger the heart rate to rise. The heart already has plenty of exercise without you even moving a muscle. Exercise is simply a more natural way to elevate the heart rate, which is why it is somewhat important. Besides, your daily activities are considered plenty of exercise your body needs for the day.

When is it a good time to exercise? The best time to exercise is in the morning before you eat breakfast, or at night before dinner because you want to exercise on an empty stomach. In order for the body to start burning the excess fat, the body needs to be empty and the body temperature must pass the equilibrium. That is why there is a saying, "running on empty." The body only burns the reserve (body fat) if the body is out of the immediate nutrients from foods and the body's temperature is above equilibrium.

Cardio

Cardio exercise is mainly to help strengthen the heart muscles. As you move, the heart beats faster to generate more blood to support the muscles exerting energy and heat. You can feel your heart beating faster as you exercise. If you continue to exercise and push the body temperature past the equilibrium, then the body will trigger the cool down process. The body will start to sweat and when wind hits the sweat, the surface of the skin will automatically cool down. Sweat occurs when the body's heat is too high and is unable to release the heat fast enough. The more you sweat, the colder the surface of your skin, the hotter you will feel. The body will continue cooling down until the heart comes to a resting rate. During this time people are accustomed to embrace the cold air which means that the body gets even colder. You will always sense heat if your surface skin's temperature is below the ambient temperature. If you want to feel cooler, use the RS Technique to raise your body temperature back up to reach equilibrium; once the surface of your skin's temperature is above the ambient temperature then you will feel cool rather than hot.

Weight training

Weight training is for individuals who want to bulk up, add some definition, or keep the body toned up. If you are planning to weight train, it is good to eat an hour before you exercise especially protein found in meat. The body needs a lot of foods to get the energy to pump iron. The heavier you lift, the more foods the body burns.

How do you know how much the body can handle? You know your body's limitation by the level of pain you are experiencing. You are pushing the body to perform at its peak, so it is dangerous and easy to push past the limitation of the body which will result in injuries. Stress marks are simply scars from torn skin tissue that have been healed by the body. The muscles outgrow the skin because the skin is not given adequate time to develop elasticity. The scar is a reminder not to push the body past its' limits. Do not ingest anything that will block the body from sensing pain like steroids because the body's only way of warning you it has reached its limit is through pain. It takes a lot of time and effort to gain muscles. The saying, "no pain, no gain" does not mean the more pain you feel the better. It simply means that you must feel the burn for the muscles to develop and grow.

Existing healing practice

For the next few chapters we will explore many healing practices and how effective they are compared to the body's system. Many healing practices assume that we understand how the body functions better than the body knows itself. We come up with different ways of treating the body, not knowing that the body needs our help, not our interference. We must first know what the body needs before we can offer our help. Otherwise, we are just interfering with the body's healing ability.

Chap. 11: Eastern healing

Eastern healing practice existed for thousands of years and it is primarily **herbal** treatment. When someone gets sick, the best place to look for a treatment is in nature. Through thousands of years of trial and error, the Chinese are well known for their extensive knowledge about herbs. They come up with many combinations of herbal formulas for different illnesses. Because herbs are nutritious like foods, it is easy to test it on humans. So their experiments advance at a quick pace. There are certainly herbs that are poisonous and many have died because of it. They were the guinea pigs of Eastern medicine. I can't say they died for a cause because Eastern herbs still lack the key factor in any cure. *The body is the only one that affects a cure.* Herbs too have ying or yang elements in them. The herbs either raise blood pressure or lower them. Take ginseng for example: it is said to have many healing properties but when you take it your heart starts to beat rapidly. It feels just like drinking alcohol. It is definitely very high in ying element.

Today herbalists draw upon ancient knowledge of herbal formulas passed down through their ancestors. For many who seek more natural treatments, herbs are the solution, but natural foods work better or just as well. Why should you pay more for herbs if your body's nutritional needs are already being met with natural foods? When a person is sick, he or she usually looses an appetite for foods. Therefore, herbs are the next best thing to give the body nutrients it needs. The herbs won't hurt you but they may affect your pocket book. Herbs in my opinion are luxury foods that are not a necessity for the body.

Another Chinese healing practice is **acupuncture.** Acupuncture consists of sticking little needles into the vein to direct blood flow. It is essentially redirecting the blood to flow to the problem area. In some cases people report improvement and others have no success. If the body is already cold and lacks blood circulation, just redirecting blood flow will not change the fact the body is cold. There are reasons why the body does what it does. No doctor or physician knows or understands why the body does what it does. This is a dangerous procedure and should only be done by a trained professional, because if performed wrong it can kill you. The blood flows a certain way for a reason and if you change the flow then you are essentially interfering with the body's natural healing process. The needle can help the body cure itself as well as cause damage to organs. Not very many acupuncturists perform this procedure even though they are trained because of liability issues.

Acupressure is very similar to acupuncture except this method is much safer and does not involve needles. Doctors massage the body's pressure points to help promote blood circulation. Putting pressure on certain veins by limiting blood flow causes the body to redirect blood to the problem area. Doctors only have one set of hands to apply the pressure and as soon as the pressure is lifted, the blood can freely flow again like it should.

There is a method called coin rubbing that my parents used on me several times when I was sick as a kid. They rubbed some menthol gel on my back and then scraped it with a coin until it turned red. It hurt like my skin was being pealed off. I guess it worked in my case because I got better as a result of it. I know my body was in shock because it sent blood to my back and I could feel the heat on my back. It may seem barbaric to some, but most Asians do not just know about it but actually use this technique every time they are sick. It is quite popular because it does not cost much and you can do it at anytime in the comfort of your home. The purpose of doing this is to promote blood circulation. (You can achieve proper blood circulation by using the pillow technique as well).

There is also another unknown method of treating the body. You start by heating up several small jars or bottles and then place it on the back. The heat builds up inside the jar to create a suction effect. Wait five to ten minutes and then remove. The suction area on your back will turn red and you can feel lots of heat on your back. This method also helps with blood circulation by forcing the body to send blood to that area. These are just a few of the Eastern healing techniques that I am aware of. I know there are many other healing techniques from other cultures. For it to be considered Eastern healing it must be natural.

Scenario 46:

You are a tough kind of guy who can handle pain. If you feel pain in your body, you just wait it out and the pain will slowly go away. You won't take any drugs and you certainly don't know any herbs to take to relieve your pain. Then your pain intensifies to a point that is unbearable.

Your friend introduces you to a doctor who performs acupuncture. You are curious enough to try. The treatment works and your pain disappears. You were pain free for a couple months, then the pain returned but you decided to stop the acupuncture treatment. It was costing too much so you just live with your pain and resort to your old method of waiting it out.

Scenario 47:

You caught the flu and your whole body is in pain. The doctor's recommendation was not to take any drugs because it raises your blood pressure. You obtained plenty of rest and drank a lot of fluid. Your fever got worse and you slept for days waking up only to use the restroom and eat. Then your mom heard you were sick, she brewed a batch of herbs and brought it over. The herbs tasted very bitter. You ask her what it is and she replied chrysanthemum tea. After drinking the tea your fever starts to die down and your pain lessens. You lay in bed longer even though you feel better because you want to be sure you are over the flu, and that it won't resurface later.

Scenario 48:

You are raised to only take herbs when you get sick. You catch a cold and can't stop coughing. You call in sick fearing others might catch it. Your mom went to the herbal store and brought home some herbs to brew. You drink the herbs and it helps out a lot. You decided to go back to work with a mild cough. The mild cough intensifies and you are now sicker than ever. Everyone at work is concerned for your health and offer all sorts of pills and remedies but none seem to work. For a week now you have been drinking the soup your mom has prepared for you. There were lots of green vegetables in the soup and a little meat. You notice the cough subsides and the workplace is quieter now that you stop coughing.

Chap 12: Western healing

Eastern herbal medicine has been the mainstream healing practice for thousands of years. However, a few hundred years ago it was replaced by Western medicine. Drugs used in Western medicine today are essentially the same as the snake oil of yesterday. Drugs are often designed for one purpose and that is to poison the body and numb the nerves so that you cannot feel the symptoms.

Drugs

Doctors with all their vast knowledge about the human body always feel they are helping the body and not interfering with the body's healing process. Every time they prescribe drugs for their patients, they cause something to happen in the body. The **law of cause and effect** can not be avoided. Everything we ingest is absorbed in the bloodstream and is carried throughout the body. How else do you expect the body to deliver the drugs to the head to numb the nerves there? The body's only means of communication is through the nervous system. By taking drugs, you are essentially numbing the bodies' only warning system (feeling). Notice how a drunk or heavily sedated person cannot feel anything but has the bruises to prove bodily harm. The abuse continues because the underlining cause of the problem is not being addressed. By numbing the nerves with drugs, the body is unable to assess the problem and warn you. Just because you don't feel pain does not mean the problem is solved. The body on drugs is essentially like a zombie. It is alive but has no sensation of pain. Take a car for example, there is an engine light to warn us that there is something wrong with the engine. Merely disconnecting the light to ignore the problem does not mean that the engine is fixed. The problem worsens as long as you ignore it and will not fix the real issue. The drugs only last a while because the body elevates the blood pressure to clean out the toxins put into the body. The body displays side effects as a way to let us know it is being abused. We get so accustomed to side effects that we are willing to sacrifice one body part for another. Destroying your liver and kidneys for the sake of suppressing pains in the body is crazy.

All drugs are made of man made chemicals which the body does not need for survival. The body is self-producing and maintains a live chemical factory. The body manufactures all the chemicals it ever needs. Any foreign chemical introduced into the body is treated as nourishment or poison. The chemicals either aid the body to heal itself or it will hurt the body by poisoning it. The body filters enough toxins from everyday foods and waste and does not need us adding more toxins into the body intentionally. Besides, the body's chemicals (cells) have intelligence and know how to self regulate unlike the static chemicals in drugs that destroy indiscriminately. Many foreign chemicals are introduced into the blood stream, it is either nutritious or poisonous to the body. Drugs are designed to mimic the body's chemicals not to replace it.

All treatments are merely providing a temporary relief and not an actual cure. Prevention is always better than treatment. We live in a fast paced society where we want everything now and have no patience whatsoever. Why do you think that fast food chains are America's number one type of restaurant? Doctors prescribe drugs to you because you can't wait for the body to heal itself and instead want instant relief. You tell the doctors to relieve you of the pain at any cost even for a short period of time. You are so happy to pay doctors to poison you. Do you know how doctors determine the dosage to prescribe to you? Doctors roughly estimate the amount of dosage to prescribe to you based on your weight and height. Notice how doctors have their nurses always measure your height and weight every visit before you see them. Based on your weight and height, your absorption rate is obtained. The higher your absorption rate, the lower your dosage is, and the lower your absorption ratio, the higher your dosage. Over the counter drugs (OTC) are no different from prescription drugs because they have the same ingredients of toxic chemicals. Prescription drugs are higher in dosage and require doctor monitoring or you may overdose on the drugs. Doctors merely determine your absorption rate so they can prescribe the dosage that will numb your nerves without killing you. You get the instant relief that you requested and all the side effects that come along with it. The body filters the drugs through the liver and kidneys and develops immunity to those drugs. That is why prolonged use of the drugs can get the body hooked on drugs. Eventually, the dosage is increased to get the numbing effect you first received using the drugs.

Shots

The most direct route of administering drugs is through intravenous injection. Instead of relying on the body's absorption rate of drugs through ingestion, the shots are usually administered in the arm into one of the veins so the blood can carry 100 % of the drugs and deliver it throughout the body. Some are administered in the buttocks for faster results since it is closest to the stomachs blood supply. The mere thought of the needle causing pain makes adults squeamish not to mention kids. As far as the body is concerned, shots are considered poison for the body. Shots are always the last resort when all other methods had failed. Why take the flu shot ahead of time when you could have saved your money and ate well enough to nourish the body so it could heal itself?

Rubs

The rub does the same thing. It too delivers the drugs by allowing the body to absorb the medication into the bloodstream through the skin. It is mainly for children who won't take their pills or get a shot, so it is the best way to administer the drugs. Either way it is all poison as far as the body is concerned. It is all designed to elevate the heart rate to produce more body heat because that is what the body really needs to repair itself. Remember that the body always raises its' temperature whenever it is bombarded with foreign chemicals. The heart will pump more blood to clean up the toxins as soon as possible.

Scenario 49:

You work and have insurance coverage through your company. You have pain now and then and every time you see your doctors, they prescribe drugs that are not covered by insurance. You are going broke because of the prescription drugs so you sometimes take OTC medicine as a replacement. You find that OTC medicine is just as effective at relieving your pain, and you spent a fraction of what you normally paid for prescription drugs. You stop going to see your doctor and continue taking OTC medicine for your pain. The money you save gives you spending money to eat out more often.

Scenario 50:

As a child, you have a fear of needles because your parent's forced you to get a shot every time you got sick, and now as an adult, you still have that fear in you. Your doctor recommends you get a shot other than oral medication because it is more effective. You finally agree to get the shot and it was over before you knew it. The only difference between the shot and the oral medication is that you become drowsy. You even lose your appetite for many days. These are a few of the many side effects you are experiencing. As soon as the medication in the shot wears off, the symptoms return in full force.

Scenario 51:

Whenever you got a stuffy nose as a kid, your parents always rubbed gel on your chest, and the vapors penetrated your nostrils to help clear your sinuses. You now use the vapor rubs yourself whenever you have sinus problems but it does not seem to work as well as when you used it as a kid. The vapor does not clear your sinuses right away so you take sinus medication along with the rub. It puts you to sleep quickly so you don't care about your sinus problems until the morning when you wake up. Then your sinuses become a nuisance as you gasp for air throughout the day.

Chap 13: Alternative heat therapies

Alternative treatments are those healing practices that are not mainstream (Eastern and Western medicine). When the two mainstream healing practices have failed, many individuals seek alternative means, but it is less popular because it is not proven to people's satisfaction. It is assumed in the healing practice that we know how to heal the body instead of the body knowing how to heal itself. We come up with all sorts of remedies that claim to cure the body but in actuality we are just helping or hurting the body's healing process. We develop massage, spa, meditation, and sauna as a way to help the body. These heat therapies all consist of one thing, and that is to aid the body to warm up and stay warm so the blood can circulate properly. These heat therapies not only help to keep the body warm but also elevate the body's metabolism to burn more efficiently.

Massage

The body is constantly under stress and needs relaxation. The tension caused by lack of body heat because of the temperature chaos condition has people seeking others to massage their body to help circulate the blood. The purpose of massage is to stimulate blood circulation to warm up the body so the muscles can relax. The body gets cold easily so instead of warming up the body yourself, you pay others to do it for you which is a waste of money and time in my opinion. People spend hundreds or even thousands of dollars for massages which you could have achieved by resting or simply applying the pillow technique when you go to sleep.

Spa

The spa treatment is another way to warm up the body and help the body relax its' tense muscles. Some believe that the constant use of the spa can help you lose weight. People believe this because they keep their body on ice all day and only when they are in the spa will the body receive heat rather than cold. It is all about keeping the blood warm so it can circulate properly. The spa is a costly treatment as well as time consuming. Your life is so hectic, how do you find time to use the spa even though you have one built in your home? You need to go to sleep anyhow, why not use the pillow technique to achieve the same thing.

Meditation

The mind is always busy thinking. Only during meditation will you remember to breathe properly. That is why meditation's main focus is on breathing. By focusing on breathing, the mind will not wander around on nonsense so the body gets a chance to relax and warm itself up. Meditation has been in existence for thousands of years as a tool for the body to reach peace and enlightenment, if you believe in such things. In my opinion, meditation is simply used to clear your mind so the body can rest. ***The body rests only if the mind rests.*** So if you have a lot of time to spare, then meditation can help you to relax mentally as well as physically. Mental relaxation is the hardest to achieve because the mind seems to have a mind of its own. It is very hard to control what you think. Nonsense often pops into your head whether you like it or not. The harder you try not to think of it, the more it surfaces in your head to taunt you. The noise around you can force you to think and distract your concentration to clear your mind. The silence around you can also contribute to your mind wandering and in effect cause you to think about unnecessary things. Mental thinking is a lengthy subject which I will discuss in detail in my future books I am planning to write.

Sauna

Saunas are no different from other heat therapy methods. Saunas are also designed to warm up the body by elevating the ambient temperature around the room past the equilibrium. Therefore, the body can sweat the fat out and detoxify the body of any toxins. The extreme heat is also used as a means to lose weight. Too much time in the sauna can cause the body to overheat because the body is unable to release its internal excess heat build up. It can cause you to collapse if the sauna room temperature is too high. Spending a lot of money and time to essentially cook yourself alive with steam instead of heat is absurd.

Remember that all these heat therapies are designed to either warm the body from the outside in by warming up the ambient temperature around the body, or to stimulate and manipulate the blood flow. The blood flow will be directed to the desired area of the body. Neither type of heat therapy lasts. The body stays warm as long as it is still in therapy. As soon as the therapy is over, the body is once again ravaged by temperature chaos.

Scenario 52:

Your job is one of those manual labor jobs that takes a great deal out of you. Your muscles are tense all the time so you and a couple of co-workers get a massage at least twice a week. The rest of the week you just put up with the discomfort because it comes with the job. You sometimes use a heating pad to warm up the area where you feel muscle tension and that helps a little. You even take painkillers to relieve (not cure) your tension. The pain seems to always linger no matter what you do.

Scenario 53:
Everyone compliments you on your beautiful figure but your opinion of yourself is different. You always watch what you eat, drink plenty of water, and exercise a lot and yet you are still not satisfied with the results. You heard that spa treatments can help you lose weight. So you get a spa treatment whenever you can afford it and can find time to go. You feel better after every spa treatment so you spend a fortune just to have your muscles relaxed.

Scenario 54:

You lose your temper easily and tend to always take it out on the wrong person. Your best friend asks you to do some meditation to calm down your temper. You did it and it relaxes your mind so your body can relax itself. Every morning you meditate for at least ten to fifteen minutes before you start your day. Everyone was surprised how calmly you handle stress. Your hot temper has died down tremendously since you practiced meditation. You tend to smile more now instead of the usual yelling.

How to take the body's temperature

Let's focus a moment on how we take the body's temperature. I have noticed that all cultures seem to respond the same way when someone is feeling sick, and that is to feel the forehead to determine if it is hot or cold. The temperature will vary depending upon the hand's temperature. Because the forehead is an extremity, relying on the forehead to determine body temperature will be inaccurate. If you want to test for the body's true temperature, you do not test the extremity (vent) but the stomach (furnace or core). Another response is to use the thermometer and test the temperature under the tongue, or worse in the rear, or the ear. Testing temperature from the ear or the rear will never get the body's true temperature reading. *Nobody knows the body better than the body knowing itself.* If you really want to test the body's temperature, the best way is to use the back of your hand between the thumb and index finger, and feel the temperature of the stomach where the naval is located. It should always stay hot. The hotter the stomach is the better. If there is extra heat it will be sent to the extremities. The cooler the stomach is, the more temperature chaos is affecting the body.

Let's recap and summarize the whole system.

- Elevate the body's temperature to reach equilibrium using the RS Technique during waking hours and the Pillow Technique during sleeping hours.

- Wear layered clothing to retain maximum body heat (equilibrium) on the stomach while the excess body heat can be released through the extremities i.e. hands, feet, and head.
- Nourish the body with natural foods from all food groups not only a select few.
- Make sure the Ying and Yang are balanced.
- Practice the Breathing Technique to help keep the blood oxygenated.
- Drink hot tea or hot drinks instead of cold drinks to help maximize the body's absorption rate and decrease waste build up in the stomach.

About the Author

Fath Saelock is a Chinese-American. Born in Laos and came to America at the age six. Fath is the middle child, "Fath in the middle" of the family. He has one older brother, one older sister, and two younger brothers. He developed this unique and revolutionary health system base upon a technique his father taught him as a child. For the last ten years, Fath, has applied the system on himself, friends, family, co-workers, and acquaintances with astounding success. Fath came to realized that the system is so safe that elderlies, kids, and even infants can use the system to stay healthy. Fath has no degree in health because the body does not certify anyone, but he does understand and listen to the body. Fath has lived up to an old saying, "physician heals thy-self".